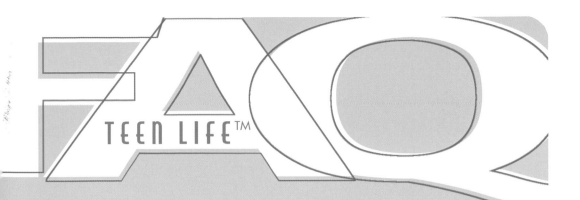

TEEN LIFE™

FREQUENTLY ASKED QUESTIONS ABOUT

# Testicular Cancer

Paula
Johanson

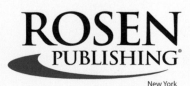

PUBLISHING®

New York

Published in 2008 by The Rosen Publishing Group, Inc.
29 East 21st Street, New York, NY 10010

First Edition

**Library of Congress Cataloging-in-Publication Data**

Johanson, Paula.
Frequently asked questions about testicular cancer / Paula
Johanson.—1st ed.
    p.cm.—(FAQ: Teen Life)
Includes bibliographical references and index.
ISBN-13: 978-1-4042-1930-4
ISBN-10: 1-4042-1930-7
1. Testis—Cancer—Popular works.
I. Title.
RC280.T4J64 2007
616.99'463—dc22

                                        2006102518

*Manufactured in the United States of America*

# Contents

# Introduction

ancer is a frightening thought for most people, particularly cancer of the reproductive organs, or genitalia. When cancer develops, an ordinary cell mutates, or changes, into an abnormal one that can't carry out its normal role in an organ. In addition, these abnormal cancerous cells divide uncontrollably, which causes a tumor to form. These tumors can, if not treated, spread quickly throughout the body and ultimately cause death. Some cancers are more aggressive and difficult to treat because of their location and resistance to chemotherapy or radiation. Fortunately, testicular cancer is very treatable when caught early. It's easy to find, and effective treatments save thousands of men's lives every year.

A monthly self-examination of your testicles (also called testes) can help you to identify tumors early, when the chance for successful treatment of testicular cancer is best. When diagnosed early, it can be combated with surgery, radiation, chemotherapy, or a combination of these treatments, depending on the type and stage of testicular cancer. If untreated, it will spread through the body and be fatal.

Testicular cancer is the most common cancer in American males between the ages of fifteen and thirty-four, but it is also one of the least mentioned cancers. Shyness about testicles doesn't give you privacy; it denies you the knowledge to keep yourself healthy. Many things contribute to silence

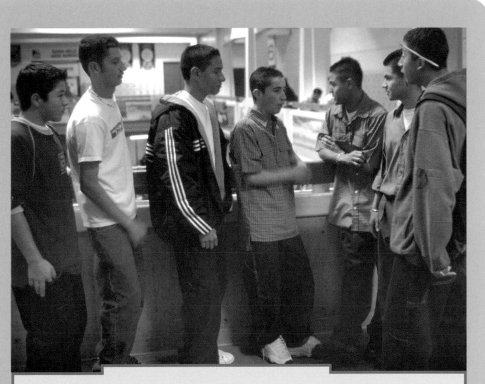

You should never be embarrassed or afraid to talk about a health problem. Testicular cancer is the most common cancer in American males between the ages of fifteen and thirty-four.

about testicular cancer—such as denial of any possible male health problem, embarrassment, ignorance, and fear. Denial will not help you. Testicular cancer is not shameful, and it is not a punishment for bad behavior. It can happen to any man. Any male health problem should be treated by a doctor, rather than ignored.

# Chapter one

## WHAT IS TESTICULAR CANCER?

Testicular cancer is a cancer that is found in one or both testicles. It accounts for about 1 percent of all cancers in males in the United States and occurs most often in males between the ages of fifteen and thirty-four. After motor vehicle accidents and suicide, testicular cancer is the third-leading cause of death for men in this age group.

In 2005, the National Cancer Institute (NCI) and the American Cancer Society (ACS) estimated that 8,000 new cases of testicular cancer were diagnosed in the United States, yet this cancer accounts for only some 380 American deaths each year. As reported by the ACS, a man's lifetime chances of getting testicular cancer is around 1 in 300. This cancer usually gets diagnosed at an early stage and is treated very successfully. According to Memorial Sloan-Kettering Cancer Center in New York City, the

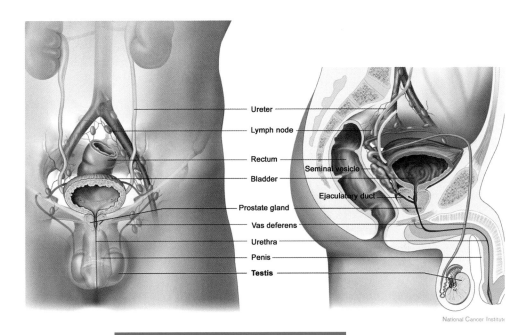

Ureter
Lymph node
Rectum
Seminal vesicle
Bladder
Ejaculatory duct
Prostate gland
Vas deferens
Urethra
Penis
**Testis**

National Cancer Institute

This illustration shows frontal and side views of the male reproductive and urinary systems. Most testicular cancers begin in the cells that produce sperm; they're called germ cell tumors.

overall cure rate for testicular cancer, when it is diagnosed early, is more than 90 percent. Celebrity survivors of this cancer include Canadian entertainer and former MTV star Tom Green and Lance Armstrong, the American professional cyclist who won the Tour de France seven consecutive times—*after* his treatment for testicular cancer. Both Green and Armstrong have spoken out about the disease and their experiences to help in destigmatizing it.

In American white men the rate of getting testicular cancer is about 4 per 100,000, while for American black men it is 1 per

# 10 FACTS ABOUT TESTICULAR CANCER

**1** If testicular cancer is treated before it spreads beyond the nearby lymph nodes, 98 percent of men live at least five years and usually a normal lifespan.

**2** Most testicular cancer is detected by the man himself.

**3** Most testicular cancer may begin as small changes in germ cells before a male was even born.

**4** Lance Armstrong won all his Tour de France bicycle races *after* surviving testicular cancer.

**5** After treatment for testicular cancer, most men are able to have erections and father children.

**6** Chemotherapy treatment for testicular cancer has improved since 1970: courses last eight to twelve weeks, instead of up to two years, and are much more effective.

**7** Radiation treatment for testicular cancer is precisely aimed at lymph nodes and is extremely effective.

**8** Testicular cancer is the most common cancer among males who are fifteen to thirty-four years old, but it's one that is rarely talked about.

**9** Some blood tests are helpful in diagnosing tumors because many testicular cancers secrete high levels of specific proteins.

**10** Good prenatal health care for women reduces future risk of testicular cancer for their sons.

100,000. The NCI estimated in 2005 that the lifetime risk for an American white man for contracting this cancer is 0.2 percent—a very low risk compared to that of prostate cancer, which may affect up to 50 percent of all men who live into their seventies.

## Your Anatomy

The testicles are two walnut-sized organs located inside the scrotum, a loose bag of skin underneath the penis. They produce male hormones (such as testosterone) and produce and store sperm for reproduction. Sperm travels from the testicle (testis) to the epididymis (coiled tubular organ), where the sperm matures, and then into the vas deferens (tubes) to the prostate gland and seminal vesicles (small glands). A nutrient-rich seminal fluid is added to a fluid from the prostate to make semen (the combined seminal fluid and sperm), which leaves the body during ejaculation. The testosterone produced by the testicles passes directly into the bloodstream.

# Tumor Types

There are three categories of testicular tumors: (1) germ cell tumors, (2) nongerm cell tumors, and (3) extragonadal tumors. Germ cell tumors are the most common and are classified as either a seminoma or a nonseminoma. Most testicular cancers start in the cells that produce the sperm and are known as germ cell tumors ("germ" means seed or sperm). Nongerm cell tumors are rare and are usually treated surgically.

The germ cells are located in tubules (tiny tubes) inside the testicles. There are two main types of germ cell testicular cancer—eminomas from immature germ cells, and nonseminomas from mature, specialized germ cells. The four histologic (having to do with the microscopic structure of tissue) classifications of non-seminomatous germ cell tumors are (1) embryonal carcinoma, (2) teratoma, (3) choriocarcinoma, and (4) yolk sac tumor. The two types of testicular cancer are treated differently, and both can be treated successfully.

The other kind of germinal cancer is stromal cell tumors, which start in the supporting tissue of the testicle. Most stromal cell tumors are benign (noncancerous) and are treated by surgery; if these tumors spread they usually do not respond to treatment.

## Categories

Doctors have named five types of germinal cancers and seven types of nongerminal cancers among all the testicular cancers. But to simplify a bit, Memorial Sloan-Kettering Cancer Center in

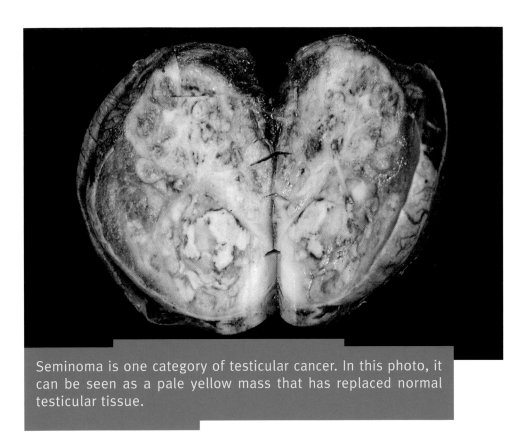

Seminoma is one category of testicular cancer. In this photo, it can be seen as a pale yellow mass that has replaced normal testicular tissue.

New York City suggests that the majority of testicular cancers can be narrowed into three categories: seminoma, nonseminoma, or some combination of the two (which are treated as nonseminomas). Their respective estimated rates of occurrence are as follows: 50 percent seminomas and 50 percent nonseminomatous germ cell tumors. Of the nonseminomas, 50 percent are embryonal carcinomas (a nonseminomatous type); 40 percent are teratoma carcinoma (a nonseminomatous type); 2 percent are choriocarcinoma (a nonseminomatous type); and 8 percent are other rare types, such as stromal cell and nongerm cell tumors.

## Most Common Types

Most testicular cancers are seminoma, embryonal carcinoma, or teratoma carcinoma. Each of these types is unique and tends to respond differently to treatment. Forbryonal carcinoma is an immature, rapidly dividing cell type. It has a tendency to metastasize (spread) earlier but is sensitive to chemotherapy or radiation therapy. Embryonal carcinoma, a type of nonsemi-nomatous germ cell tumor, is rarely treated with radiation therapy. Teratoma carcinoma, a mixture of teratoma and embryonal carcinoma, is less sensitive to radiation but very sensitive to chemotherapy. Teratomas are germ cell tumors with areas that, when viewed with a microscope, resemble each of the three layers of a developing embryo.

Seminoma is the most common testicular cancer in the age group of thirty- to forty-year-olds. About 85 percent of men who get testicular cancer have this type. It is a well-differentiated tumor cell, and in about 15 percent of cases there are other trophoblastic cell elements (misshaped cells that can be seen with a microscope) present. These produce a version of the hormone human chorionic gonadotropin (beta HCG). This allows doctors to monitor for the progress of the disease as it is being treated by watching the HCG levels in the blood.

## Secondary Tumors

Secondary testicular tumors are those that start in another organ and then spread to the testicle. Lymphoma is the most common secondary testicular cancer. Among men older than fifty, testicular lymphoma is more common than primary testicular tumors.

## Stages of Cancer

Once testicular cancer has been diagnosed by a doctor, the doctor needs to determine how far the cancer has spread. The process in which tests are used to make this determination and help doctors decide the course of treatment is called staging. The staging of testicular cancer can be complex, but it is usually described as being in Stage 0, Stage I, Stage II, or Stage III. Stage 0 is also known as carcinoma in situ (CIS) and is the stage where abnormal cells are confined within the testicle and have not spread. Stage I is divided into two subcategories: Stage IA and Stage IB. The subcategory is determined after the affected testicle has been removed in surgery. In Stage IA, the tumor marker levels in the patient's blood are normal, but the cancer has perhaps spread to the tissue around the testicle. In Stage IB, the cancer has spread from the testicle to the lymph system or the blood, the surrounding tissue, or the scrotum. Stage II is when the cancer is in the testicle, spermatic cord, or scrotum, and has spread to some of the lymph nodes behind the peritoneum; this stage is called Bulky Stage II when more than five lymph nodes are swollen greater than three-quarters of an inch across. In Nonbulky Stage II, the cancer is within the testicle, spermatic cord, or scrotum, and has spread to up to five abdominal lymph nodes, but the lymph nodes have not swollen larger than three-quarters of an inch. In Stage III, the cancer has spread beyond the retroperitoneal lymph nodes. In Nonbulky Stage III, the cancer is confined to the lymph nodes and the lungs, and a single tumor is no greater in size than three-quarters of an inch. In Bulky Stage III, the cancer has spread to multiple areas within the body, including the lymph nodes, with tumors that are bigger than three-quarters of an inch, and to organs other than the lungs.

# Genetic Alteration

The cells that make up your body each have forty-six chromosomes in the nucleus, arranged in twenty-three pairs. These chromosomes contain genes that are a plan for everything in your body, coded in long molecules of deoxyribonucleic acid (DNA). Small changes in the DNA happen by accident all the time. Some of these changes can lead to the cell not being able to function properly as a germ cell (or liver cell, or whatever kind it is). Usually your immune system detects this cell and gets rid of it. These cancer cells can multiply and grow. Some kinds of cancer multiply quickly and spread through the bloodstream or lymph system to other organs.

Testicular germ cell tumors show characteristic changes: gains at chromosome pairs 7, 8, 12, 21, and X and losses at chromosome pairs 11, 13, and 18. About 80 percent of testicular tumors have specific alterations to the twelfth chromosome pair. It may be that a third of all cases of testicular cancer are in men who carry a recessive gene that makes this cancer more possible when they are exposed to the right conditions.

# Cryptorchidism

Since the 1850s, doctors have known that males who have undescended testicles (at birth, one or both testes remain inside the abdomen instead of descending into the scrotum), a condition called cryptorchidism, are at higher risk for testicular cancer. The risk is ten to forty times greater—still only about 4 in 10,000 for American white men. Even with this higher risk for males with cryptorchidism, 95 percent of testicular cancers occur in males whose testicles descended normally. Although only 2 percent of testicular cancers occur in both testes, about 50 percent of those that do are in patients with cryptorchidism.

# Carcinoma in Situ (CIS)

The types of testicular cancers that commonly occur in men are preceded by atypical intratubular germ cells called carcinoma in situ, or CIS. (*Carcinoma in situ* is Latin for "cancer in place," a cancer that doesn't grow or spread.) The cell changes may have happened when the male was a fetus or baby. These changes may be much more common in germ cells left behind when the testicles develop and descend into the scrotum. It's possible to have a germ cell carcinoma that begins in the lower abdominal lymph nodes behind the peritoneum, instead of inside a testicle.

Doctors don't do random testing for CIS. Nobody is sure how rare or common CIS may be, or how often it develops into testicular cancer. It's hard to do animal studies on the causes for testicular cancer because CIS is extremely rare in laboratory animals.

This photomicrograph shows human X *(right)* and Y *(left)* sex chromosomes. Chromosomes contain the genetic material DNA, in which small changes can lead to germ cells not being able to function properly. Testicular germ cell tumors typically show gains at chromosome pairs 7, 8, 12, 21, and X and losses at pairs 11, 13, and 18.

Testicular cancer is usually detected by the man himself, rather than by a doctor. The most common way it becomes manifest is as a painless testicular mass. A lump may be found by accident or during a doctor's routine physical examination. A doctor is easily able to tell through tests if a lump is a tumor. Don't be afraid to ask your doctor any question, no matter how simple you may think it is. If you have any signs or symptoms of a tumor, consult with your doctor.

# Chapter two

## HOW IS TESTICULAR CANCER DETECTED AND DIAGNOSED?

### How to Do a Self-Exam

Monthly testicular self-examinations are recommended after puberty, especially for males at increased risk for testicular cancer. Finding tumors early increases the chance for curing this form of cancer.

The best time to examine your testicles is during or after a warm bath or shower, when the skin of the scrotum is relaxed. Examine each testicle gently with both hands. Place the index and middle fingers underneath the testicle, and place the thumbs on top. Roll the testicle gently between the thumbs and fingers.

The testicles should be smooth, oval, and rather firm. One testicle may feel a little larger than the other. This is normal. If one changes to become larger, this is abnormal. You will feel something like a cord on the top

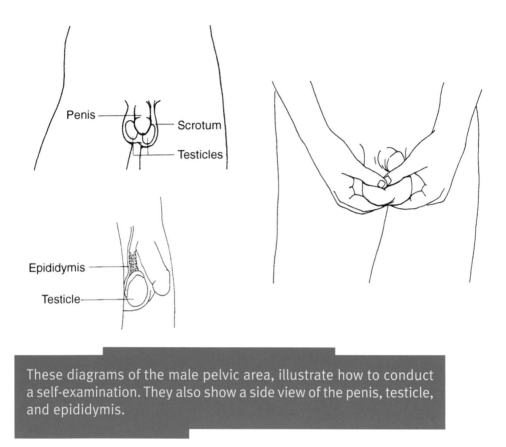

These diagrams of the male pelvic area, illustrate how to conduct a self-examination. They also show a side view of the penis, testicle, and epididymis.

and back of each testicle. This is the epididymis, the organ that stores and transports the sperm, not an abnormal lump.

If you find an abnormal lump, hard or soft, on either testicle or in the scrotum, visit your doctor within a week maximum—or right away if you have pain. The doctor will examine you thoroughly, checking for signs of swelling. The doctor will also check your abdomen to see if your lymph nodes are enlarged. If the lump is caused by an infection, a cyst, or an injury, it will be treated and will heal. The doctor will do tests to determine if the lump is a tumor.

# Common Symptoms of Testicular Cancer

More than 90 percent of men with testicular cancer find a painless lump or mass in the testicle. It is usually hard and can be as small as a grain of rice. Sometimes a testicle may feel swollen, larger, or shaped differently from the other testicle.

There may be discomfort or pain in a testicle or the scrotum in 10 percent of the cases. Some men may also notice a sensation of heaviness in the scrotum or a dull ache in the groin, lower back, or lower abdomen. Or they may feel a lump in the neck if the cancer has spread.

Scrotal enlargement or swelling is common in those with testicular cancer. It may feel like fluid is collecting in the scrotum.

In about 5 percent of the cases, hormonal changes will cause a man's breasts to swell or his nipples to become tender. Other hormonal changes might make facial and body hair much coarser and thicker than would be expected for a male in his teens.

# Don't Ignore It, But Don't Panic

Don't panic if you have any of these symptoms! It may be for other health reasons, which are also worth looking into. See a doctor if any of these symptoms last a week—sooner if you have pain. Early treatment solves many health problems easily, and early treatment is the best thing for testicular cancer, which can double in size in a month.

Many of these symptoms can be caused by a testicle injury or infection. Other symptoms can be caused by a bladder infection or hernia, which can be treated. Even sore nipples might be due only to wearing a rough shirt while jogging. It makes sense to get help for any health problem and to be confident whether or not your symptom is caused by cancer.

Consult your doctor if you have any of the following symptoms:

- Lump or mass in either testicle
- Enlargement or swelling of a testicle
- Collection of fluid or a swelling in the scrotum
- Dull ache in the groin, lower abdomen, or back
- Feeling of heaviness in the scrotum
- Discomfort or pain in a testicle or in the scrotum
- Enlargement or tenderness of the breast and nipple areas

## Blood Tests

Blood tests can detect some important tumor markers. Alpha-fetoprotein tests positive for some men with testicular cancer and can be used to monitor for remissions (the tumors are gone) or relapses (the tumors have recurred). Beta HCG can also test positive, as it does when females have choriocarcinoma. Another substance to test for is lactate dehydrogenase (LDH).

## Other Tests

The doctor will confirm that this is not any other condition, such as fluid accumulation in a testicle (hydrocele), sperm-filled cyst

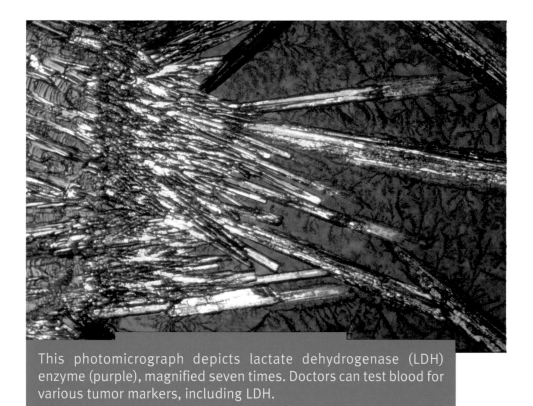

This photomicrograph depicts lactate dehydrogenase (LDH) enzyme (purple), magnified seven times. Doctors can test blood for various tumor markers, including LDH.

(spermatocele), enlarged veins (variocele), inflammation of a testicle (orchitis), or twisting of the testicle (torsion). Lymphoma (cancer of the lymph nodes) will also have to be ruled out.

Any man with a testicular mass will need a scrotal ultrasound, which will help differentiate between the other conditions listed above. In addition, a man with testicular cancer may need CT scans (computerized axial tomography, a detailed form of X-ray picture) of the abdomen and pelvis and a chest X-ray. If the chest X-ray is abnormal, then the doctor may order a CT of the chest. Other exams may need to be ordered as indicated, for example, a CT of the man's head.

Possibly MRI (magnetic resonance imagery) scans or PET (positron emission tomography) scans of other structures may be ordered to see if the cancer is in any of these places. All of these locations can harbor germ cells from before the man was born, cells that can degenerate into cancer.

# three

# HOW IS TESTICULAR CANCER TREATED?

You might receive one type of treatment, or a combination of treatments, depending on the type of testicular cancer that you have and the stage to which it has progressed. The three main types of treatment are surgery, chemotherapy, and radiation therapy. There are many things you can do to help yourself feel better during treatment and recovery. A positive attitude is something that is crucial to your health. Plan to get better and resume normal activities, and plan to have regular checkups every year afterward.

## Preparing Yourself for Surgery

Before surgery, you may be asked to wash your genitals thoroughly with a soft scrub brush, and an electric clipper may be used in the operating room right before surgery

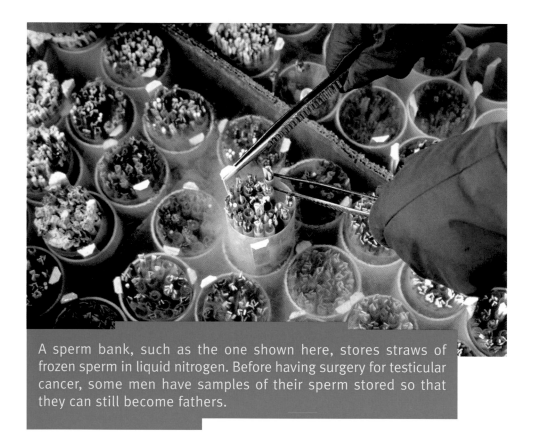

A sperm bank, such as the one shown here, stores straws of frozen sperm in liquid nitrogen. Before having surgery for testicular cancer, some men have samples of their sperm stored so that they can still become fathers.

to clip your pubic hair. When the pubic hair grows back later, the sprouting hairs will feel sharp and some might be ingrown or inflamed. There are over-the-counter creams that minimize this irritation. Before long, your pubic hair will return to its natural growth.

Before surgery, you may want to store a sample of your sperm at a sperm bank. Men who have had one testicle removed can still become fathers. However, you may appreciate having your sample available if needed. The more important reason for banking sperm is that the chemotherapy regimen used to treat some forms of testicular cancer can cause infertility.

Ask the doctor to test your testosterone count before surgery. If it turns out that you need hormone therapy later on, it's good to know what "normal" was for you.

Ask your doctor if he or she plans to use staples or dissolving sutures when closing the incision. Some doctors recommend one over the other. Some patients have had other surgery before and can inform the doctor on which method was used then and how it felt as it healed. Advise your doctor if the scar feels painful or numb, and how this changes during healing.

Some people recommend avoiding funny movies and jokes for a couple of days after surgery. Laughing can hurt! But a week or so later, humor can be an important part of the process of feeling better.

# Orchiectomy

The surgery will be done under either a general or a local anesthetic, and it takes about an hour. You will probably stay in the hospital overnight.

Most of the time, the entire testicle is removed (orchiectomy) with the cord, not just the tumor. Your doctor will not schedule a biopsy first to take a sample of the tumor for study as is done for some other cancers. The tumor will be examined very carefully during your surgery to see if it is malignant (spreading), but very few tumors of the testicles are benign (not likely to grow much or spread).

The incision for the orchiectomy will be in your groin, not your scrotum. When it heals, the scar will be mostly hidden in your pubic hair.

# Ten Great Questions to Ask When You're Asking for Help

**1** Does this testicular cancer mean I'm going to die soon?

**2** What experts are we going to consult?

**3** Can you give me anything to read about this cancer and its treatments?

**4** What cancer treatments do you recommend?

**5** What if I want to father children in the future?

**6** Can you test my hormone levels before cancer treatment?

**7** If my testicle is removed, can I have a fake one put in so my scrotum looks like it used to?

**8** What should I be telling you about how my healing process feels after surgery?

**9** Is there anyone I can talk to about surviving cancer, maybe in a self-help group?

**10** Does my having testicular cancer mean male relatives will get it, too?

# Retroperitoneal Lymph Node Dissection

A retroperitoneal lymph node dissection (RPLND) is done when a CT scan shows that cancer has spread to the lymph nodes behind the peritoneum in the lower abdomen, or if the microscopic analysis of the testicle shows that the cancer has invaded the blood or lymphatic vessels. The peritoneum is a membrane that holds your abdominal organs in place. The intestines will be moved aside so the lymph nodes behind the peritoneum can be removed. The space behind the peritoneum, around the kidneys, will be examined as well. The surgery takes about four to six hours and is done under a general anesthetic.

It's important to avoid becoming constipated after abdominal surgery. Codeine does reduce pain, but it is constipating. You may find that drinking prune juice, taking Metamucil (a powdered fiber mixed in water), or prescription laxatives is enough to keep your bowels moving.

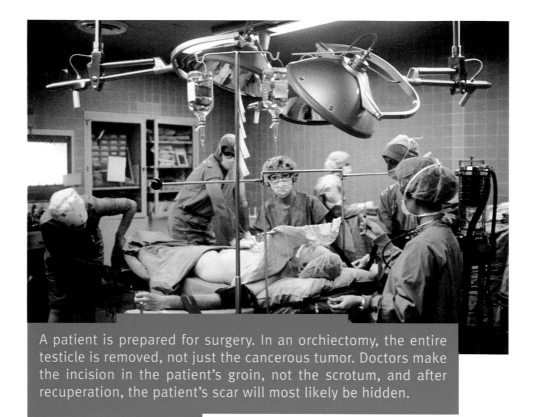

A patient is prepared for surgery. In an orchiectomy, the entire testicle is removed, not just the cancerous tumor. Doctors make the incision in the patient's groin, not the scrotum, and after recuperation, the patient's scar will most likely be hidden.

# Preparing Yourself for Chemotherapy

Chemotherapy is the use of drugs for treating cancer. You may have hair loss from chemotherapy—ask your doctor if this is likely with your medication. Many people prefer to be in control and cut their hair short or buzz it all off, rather than wait until it falls out in clumps. A haircut is less of a shock to yourself and to others. Your hair will grow back after a couple of months and may be a slightly different color or texture. Don't be alarmed if your body hair falls out, too.

Chemotherapy reduces your white blood cell count and may make you more susceptible to infection, including tooth problems. See your dentist before beginning treatment because having a dental abscess treated or getting teeth pulled during a course of chemotherapy is pain that can be avoided. Use a mouthwash before and throughout chemotherapy. Sucking on ice cubes relieves pain and also keeps the mouth moist. Mouth sores are another side effect of chemotherapy.

## Drugs Used in Chemotherapy

The drugs prescribed in chemotherapy may be used alone or in combinations. They include cisplatin (Platinol), bleomycin (Blenoxane), vinblastine (Velban), cyclophosphamide (Cytoxan), etoposide (Etopophos), and ifosfamide (Ifex). Side effects of their use may include gastrointestinal disturbances, low blood count, skin disorders, and neurological disorders. The newer class of drugs are endonuclease inhibitors: for example, Ukrain, which is still being studied in Germany and Russia. Ask your doctor if your chemotherapy drugs may have long-term effects on your health.

## Delivery of Treatment

Each treatment will take a couple of hours, during which you can nap, read, or watch television. Some people meditate or pray and visualize the treatment working. Others think about something else. The medication will be delivered into a vein in your arm, which may be given a port (membrane liner) to minimize irritation from repeated treatments every few days

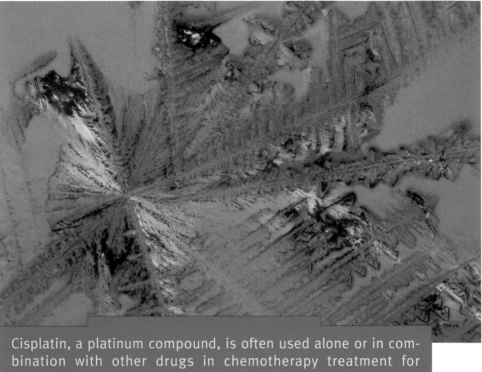

Cisplatin, a platinum compound, is often used alone or in combination with other drugs in chemotherapy treatment for testicular cancer. Side effects from chemotherapy may include gastrointestinal problems, low blood count, skin disorders, and neurological disorders.

or once each week. Massage can help your arms feel better afterward.

The chemicals you are given will have the strongest effect upon rapidly dividing cells, like cancer and the hair-growing cells. You may not have any negative effects at all, but many people feel weak or tired during the next day or two. There may be an odd taste in your mouth; lemonade or pineapple juice may rinse this taste away. Some kinds of food may not taste good and you might not have much of an appetite.

# Preparing Yourself for Radiation

Radiation therapy is used to treat seminomas. In radiation therapy, a beam of high-energy X-rays is used to destroy cancerous cells or retard their rate of growth. Ask your doctor if you should expect hair loss or if you need to see the dentist before beginning radiation treatments, just as you do when preparing for chemotherapy. Ask if you will have enough radiation to worry about exposing someone you sleep beside.

## Delivery of Treatment

Radiation from the high-energy X-rays will be aimed at the lymph nodes in your lower abdomen. Because this treatment usually follows an orchiectomy, your remaining testicle will be carefully shielded to protect it. The technicians will tattoo small marks on your skin to ensure that the radiation is aimed precisely. These small marks will fade in time. Each treatment will take a couple of minutes, every few days or once a week, or possibly less frequently. Some people meditate or pray and visualize the treatment working, while others think about something else.

Radiation will have the most effect on the lymph nodes, where it is aimed. You may feel tired or weak for the next day or two. It's possible that you will have diarrhea and your skin will feel sunburned. You might not have much of an appetite because of nausea. Eat what tastes good to you.

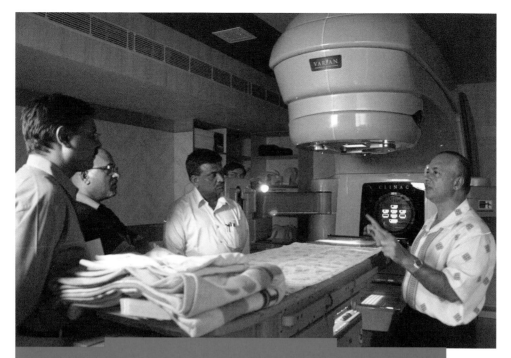

In radiation therapy for testicular cancer, high-energy X-rays are aimed at the lymph nodes in a patient's lower abdomen. Each treatment usually takes a couple of minutes every few days or perhaps once per week, depending on the course of treatment.

## Carrying a Note

Carry a note from your doctor indicating that you are receiving radiation treatments. The note should have a phone number where someone may be contacted to confirm your therapy. You may set off radiation detectors at an airport or customs department, and the officials will need to know why.

# Nausea

Many people go through an entire course of chemotherapy or radiation treatments and never feel nauseated. But for others, nausea is perhaps the most upsetting factor.

The easiest way to avoid nausea is by drinking lots of water every day. Don't get dehydrated! Drink at least eight glasses of water every day, and tea or fruit juice as well. Eating ginger or drinking ginger tea works to settle the stomach. Some people prefer drinking black tea, green tea, or herbal tea.

Other treatments for nausea include acupuncture (a Chinese medical treatment in which needles are placed at several points on the body), acupressure (pressure with fingertips at acupuncture points), and wearing a wristband that presses on an acupressure point. Try mild exercise before or after the treatment.

Diet is a big factor in whether or not you get nauseated. Avoid greasy and highly spiced foods. Try a variety of foods to find some that don't upset your stomach. You may end up making nutritious fruit milkshakes and smoothies to replace some meals.

Be willing to take antinausea medication prescribed by your doctor, perhaps starting before the treatment begins.

# Improved Treatments

Treatments for testicular cancer have improved a great deal during the past thirty years. Diagnostic X-rays, ultrasound exams, CT scans, PET scans, and MRIs can detect with pinpoint accuracy if cancer cells have spread elsewhere in the body.

Fruit smoothies can be a nutritious meal for someone who is having problems with nausea after chemotherapy or radiation treatments. Eat what tastes good to you, if you have an upset stomach.

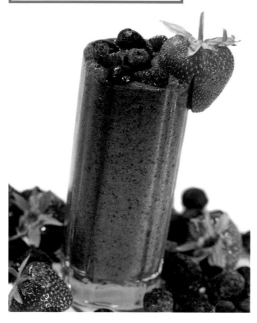

Surgical techniques are much more delicate, so nerve damage is less likely and incisions heal neater with less pain. After an orchiectomy, a man's remaining testicle is shielded from radiation treatment so that he continues to have not only a natural source of testosterone, but also remain fertile. Radiation is now delivered in lower doses and is precisely aimed. Chemotherapy during the 1970s used to take up to two years, but now regimens have been developed that take only twelve to sixteen weeks to complete. There are new drug treatment protocols being developed, and research proceeds also into increasingly delicate surgical techniques (such as stem cell research).

Survivors can expect that after treatments, they will recover their good health and a sense of well-being. Strength and vigor will return with good nutrition and exercise—and a good attitude. Some survivors have gone on to begin or resume careers as professional athletes or competitors at the

Olympic Games. Hormone treatment can be given to men who have had one or both testicles removed, often using patches for a slow, steady release of the hormones—the dosage will be carefully adjusted for the best outcome.

## Increasing Survival

Back in the 1970s, the five-year survival rate (meaning that the person is alive five years after diagnosis) for testicular cancer was only 10 percent. But due to increased awareness, early detection, radiation treatments, and chemotherapy, the survival rate is now more than 90 percent. If the cancer has not spread to the lymph nodes, 98 percent of cases can be cured. Most survivors now lead long, normal lives afterward and get yearly checkups. Such success stories begin with every male doing regular self-exams.

## WHO IS AT RISK FOR DEVELOPING TESTICULAR CANCER?

Anything that increases a person's chance of having a disease is called a risk factor. No one is certain what causes testicular cancer, or how to prevent it from happening to one man or to any group of men. But researchers are proposing ideas that may reduce the risk for future generations. However, if you have a risk factor for testicular cancer, that does not mean you will contract the disease.

### Age

Young men have a higher risk of getting testicular cancer than elderly men. This is the most common cancer for men between the ages of twenty and thirty-four, the second-most common in men between the ages of thirty-five and thirty-nine, and the third-most common in men between the ages of fifteen to nineteen. It's rare

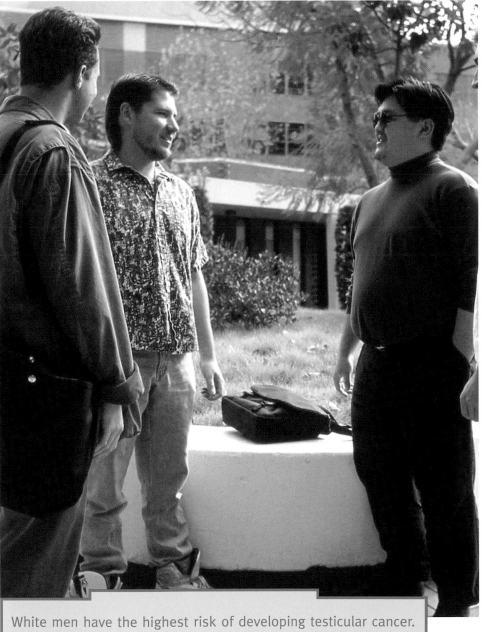

White men have the highest risk of developing testicular cancer. Hispanic, Asian, and Native American men are more likely to be at risk than black men, but not as likely as white men.

# Myths and Facts

## About Testicular Cancer

**If I have cancer in my genitals, I can never father children.** Fact ●➤ Most men who have had one testicle removed can father children. You can choose to store your semen in a sperm bank before surgery. Remember that adoptive fathers and stepfathers are real dads, too!

**I can't get testicular cancer because I never had a sexually transmitted disease.** Fact ●➤ Testicular cancer is not caused by sexually transmitted diseases.

**One of my testicles was undescended, so I'll definitely get cancer there.** Fact ●➤ Males with an undescended testicle are ten to forty times more likely to get testicular cancer, but the lifetime risk is still only about 2 percent. A blood test and monthly self-exams are all the extra worry this is worth.

**I'm not a real man if I don't have both testicles.**
Fact ➡ Manhood is in your mind as well as in your body. If hormone replacement therapy is needed, your doctor will help you with that.

**Riding a bicycle causes testicular cancer.** Fact ➡
Bike riding does not cause any cancer; it promotes good health. A hard bike seat may press on a nerve and cause numbness or temporary impotence. To avoid this, use a comfortable seat with a gel or sheepskin seat cover, or try a recumbent bike.

for men aged forty to sixty, but after age sixty there are a few cases. Testicular cancer can affect males of any age.

## Race

Testicular cancer is most common among white men. Hispanic, Asian, and Native American men are more likely than black men to develop testicular cancer, but not as likely as white men. Men of all races should still do monthly self-exams.

## Family History

If a family member has testicular cancer, you have an increased risk for developing it as well. If your mother was prescribed DES (diethylstilbestrol) during her pregnancy with you, you have an increased risk. DES is a synthetic female hormone that was intended to reduce a pregnant woman's chance of a miscarriage, but it is no longer used. Certainly you should do monthly self-exams and have your blood tested.

## Personal History

If you've already had testicular cancer, you have a higher risk of developing it in the other testicle. You also have a higher risk of developing other cancers. Expect to have cancer check-ups every year for the rest of your life.

Men with undescended testicles have an increased risk of testicular cancer, even if the undescended testicle has been surgically moved to the scrotum. There are congenital (existing at birth) conditions that increase a man's risk of testicular cancer, such as gonadal dysgenesis (being born with a Y chromosome change, which means the testes did not form normally) or Klinefelter's syndrome (being born with at least two X chromosomes as well as at least one Y chromosome, instead of an XY pair like most males).

Having a vasectomy does not increase a man's risk of getting testicular cancer. During a vasectomy, the vas deferens are cut and tied, making a man sterile but still potent (able to have erections). Doctors are researching whether having a vasectomy might increase the rate at which an existing, but undetected, testicular cancer will progress. About one man in six over the age of thirty-five chooses a vasectomy for birth control, and he is more likely to be health-conscious and do self-exams.

## Location

The percentage of men who develop testicular cancer shows marked geographic variation. For instance, the incidence is higher in Europe than on other continents, and it is also higher among northern Europeans than central or southern Europeans. The highest rate of testicular cancer in Europe is in Denmark, where each year there are now 7.8 cases diagnosed per 100,000 men. In China and Japan, and for people of African descent around the world, the rate is about 1 per 100,000 men.

As nations become more affluent, the rate of men diagnosed with testicular cancer increases. Since 1940 in Western nations, the number of European men diagnosed with this cancer each year has been increasing by 2 percent annually. Increased socioeconomic status affects what a person eats and what exposure to pollution he or she may experience; this has an effect on many kinds of cancer.

## Exposure in Infancy

Because testicular cancer is most prevalent among young men between the ages of fifteen and thirty-four, the statistics suggest this is due to exposure to something either in the womb or early in life. This exposure may damage DNA in testicular cells in a fetus or baby boy.

Some researchers believe that exposure to ochratoxin A during early childhood or before birth may set up the testes so that hormonal changes and testicular growth during puberty and maturity trigger the beginning of testicular cancer. Ochratoxin A is a common carcinogen in mold that grows in grains and coffee beans and is found in animals that eat moldy grain, especially pigs. When pregnant women and nursing mothers eat foods with ochratoxin A, this carcinogen is present in their blood and milk. It's too small an amount to have much effect on an adult, but it may affect the rapidly growing cells in fetuses and babies.

If this theory is true, what can anyone do to reduce the risk of exposing a fetus or baby to ochratoxin A? Weather conditions during grain harvests may lead to moldy grain. Even certified organically raised grains, coffee beans, and pork could still have tiny amounts of ochratoxin A. Danish people eat more pork per capita than almost any other nation, and they also eat the most rye, the cereal grain that is most often contaminated by ochratoxin A. If this is a factor in their higher rate of testicular cancer, it will be challenging to make dietary changes as a nation.

Some researchers recommend that vitamins A, C, and E should be taken by pregnant women to reduce the toxicity of ochratoxin A. Fortunately, most pregnant and nursing women are advised by their doctors to eat foods containing these vitamins and to take dietary supplements as well.

## Estrogen Overexposure

Estrogen is a necessary hormone for males and females, but a fetus might be overexposed to estrogen in the womb, which can cause damage to testicular DNA. Doctors prescribe hormone therapies—even the birth control pill—very carefully to women of childbearing age to avoid this risk. DES, a synthetic form of

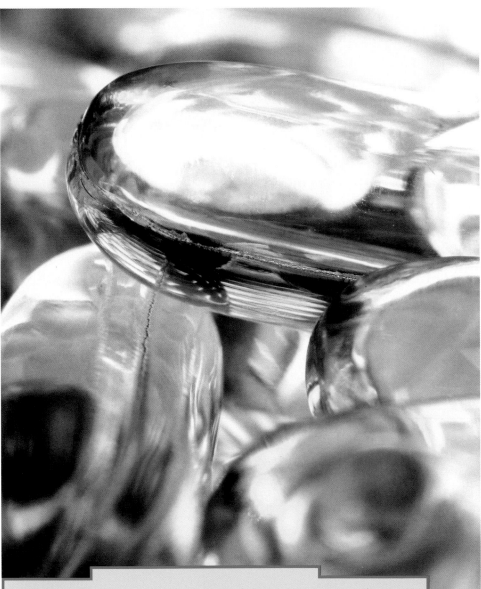

Some medical research has indicated that exposure to ochratoxin A before birth or in early childhood can trigger the beginning of testicular cancer. A number of researchers recommend that pregnant women take vitamins A, C, and E, which is seen here, to reduce the toxicity of ochratoxin A.

estrogen, is no longer prescribed for pregnant women because their sons have an increased risk of testicular cancer and their daughters have an increased risk of female health problems.

In addition, because commercially sold milk is now produced from pregnant cows, milk and dairy products contain some female sex hormones such as estrogen and progesterone. Also, a significant elevated risk of testicular cancer has been linked to exposure to polyvinyl chloride; this and other "plastic" materials release estrogen-mimic chemicals into food and water. These exposures to pregnant women in general may increase the risk when combined with individual experiences such as pollution, or genetic factors that researchers haven't learned to recognize.

# five

# HOW WILL TESTICULAR CANCER AFFECT MY LIFESTYLE?

It's hard to think that there is good news about having cancer of any kind. But honestly, this form of cancer is detectable early by ordinary people as well as doctors. The tests for it are reliable. The treatments work very effectively, especially when the cancer is detected at an early or moderate stage.

Cancer survivors often report that they no longer take life for granted, and that they receive great satisfaction from achieving their goals for their work and home lives. Accomplishing things you've always hoped to do can mean a lot more when you've survived cancer.

## A Healthy Lifestyle

There are many things you can do to improve your general health. Don't smoke or use any tobacco products, solve

You can improve your general health by choosing physical activity such as running, not smoking tobacco products, and eating a well-balanced diet, among other things.

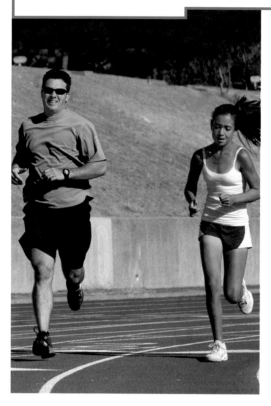

problems that are causing you stress, and be physically active every day. During cancer treatment you may find that yoga stretches and a short walk are all you can do for a few days. Gradually increase your daily activity till you are spending an hour or more having a brisk walk, playing sports, or doing physical work.

Your diet should consist mainly of fresh vegetables and fruit, and whole grains. Avoid deli meats and highly processed foods; instead, eat fish for a good source of protein and vitamins. Drink five or six glasses of water every day, and no more than one cup of coffee. Adults should have no more than one drink of alcohol in a day.

A healthy lifestyle will not only help your treatments work and your strength return, it will also reduce your risk of another cancer diagnosis in the future.

During cancer treatment, engage in physical activity slowly. Once your strength returns, participate in sports such as crew, or some other exercise to help you improve your health and mental attitude.

## Self-Help Groups

For some men, it doesn't seem manly to talk about health problems or emotions at all. But medical treatment alone is not enough. Sooner or later, you will either want to talk with people who understand what you are experiencing—or you will be fed up with people who don't have a clue.

Other people who are surviving cancer can give you a lot of support that really helps because they've been through the same things you are facing. It can help to know that you are not the only one who feels the way you do. A self-help group can be very relaxed and casual, and you can study a series of readings together. You don't have to go through psychotherapy or have a big emotional breakthrough. Some groups meet at community buildings a few times each year or once per month. If your community has no self-help or support group at present, consult your nurses about setting one up. You might also join a self-help group on the Internet or post messages on an Internet list server or chat room. Even though online support groups can be helpful, they should never be a substitute for getting professional psychological and medical care. You should always visit your doctor first. Moreover, when you meet people online, make sure you use good judgment. Don't give out personal information such as your address or telephone number. Make sure your username doesn't accidentally reveal that information. Never agree to meet someone face to face without checking with your parents first and getting their approval. Be sure that you meet in a public place and take a friend with you. Tell your parents who you are meeting and when and where you are meeting. Be careful when looking for online groups and make sure that you research information that you get online because sometimes it can be inaccurate.

## Positive Attitude

Looking forward to renewed good health, making plans for the future, feeling a sense of hope, and making the best of things—these are all part of having a positive attitude. It's no substitute for treatment, but it works well with modern medicine to improve survival rates and quality of life. You may find that prayer or meditation helps you, as well as sports and art and studies. Some men decide they'd better have a positive attitude because they plan to live many decades and not be upset by having to get tested every year or so for cancer.

Keeping a sense of humor is a way of being in charge of your feelings and attitudes, even when you are going through treatments. Many Web sites for survivors of testicular cancer include a page of jokes on the topic. This cheerful and raunchy humor is one option to help you maintain a positive attitude.

## Family Ought to Know

If you have been diagnosed with testicular cancer, your male relatives are at a higher risk than the general population. Don't feel any guilt about this. Just make sure that each of them—and your male friends—knows to do a monthly self-exam and get tested for testicular cancer on a regular basis. Maybe you could get pamphlets for them to read, or make your own by printing a page from the Internet. You could write a short, serious note or a funny cartoon, and make photocopies to give them. Even your female friends and relatives may be interested so they can help the men in their lives look after their own health.

Your family deserves to know so they will understand what's happening to you. Everyone cares about the people in their lives and wants to do anything that may help. Maybe you don't need their help or even a ride to the treatment center—but at least now you won't get asked to paint the kitchen or go waterskiing two days after surgery. You're more likely to get the reactions you want from your family if you thank them for caring and tell them what you do need.

# Your Sexual Feelings

A few men diagnosed with testicular cancer find that their sexual feelings are affected for a while. That's natural. Some of that is just from having any health problem at all. Some of that is from having been diagnosed with cancer—a life-threatening condition. And some may be from how you feel about having cancer in your genitals. It will usually get better as your sense of well-being returns. Be willing to talk about how your feelings are affected, perhaps maybe with your self-help group or a therapist. Your doctor might test your hormones.

## Retrograde Ejaculation

After an orchiectomy, most men with one testicle will continue to produce sperm. For a few men, after an RPLND, ejaculation will release semen into the bladder instead of out the penis. This condition is called retrograde ejaculation. In these cases, men are still able to have erections and orgasms but are less likely to father a child. New surgical techniques can prevent the nerve damage causing this problem.

# Can Anyone Tell?

No one can tell by looking at you that you have testicular cancer. This cancer doesn't make you look, talk, or behave differently. When the incision from your surgery heals, the scar can be covered

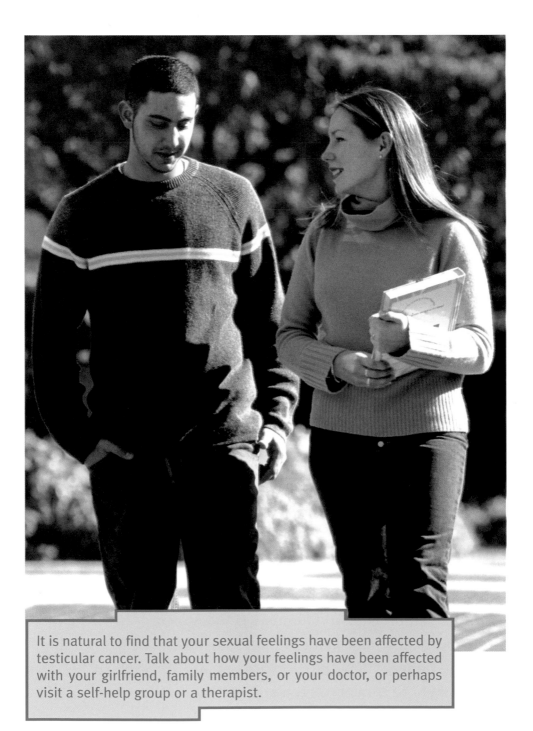

It is natural to find that your sexual feelings have been affected by testicular cancer. Talk about how your feelings have been affected with your girlfriend, family members, or your doctor, or perhaps visit a self-help group or a therapist.

by a bathing suit. The scar will be in or near your pubic hair, and it will usually be difficult to see.

If you have an orchiectomy, your scrotum may not look much different. Generally, no one would be able to tell from a casual glance if you are naked in the shower at a gym, for example. Some men choose to have a molded silicone shell that is filled with saline implanted as an artificial testicle. This testicular prosthesis is placed inside the scrotum during later surgery. This prosthesis will look and feel much like a real testicle. These silicone implants, which are filled with saline (saltwater) have all the same medical concerns as silicone breast implants for women, so it's not a decision to make casually.

# Speaking Out About Testicular Cancer

It can be hard to talk about your genitalia at first, even to a doctor or someone who cares about you. But if you tell people that you have cancer, some of them may ask what kind. It's up to you to decide how much you will tell any particular person about your health. You do not have to be the spokesman for testicular cancer. Just be able to say a little when you think it is important.

## Tom Green

Canadian entertainer and former MTV actor Tom Green survived testicular cancer and made a one-hour television special about his experience, including footage of his surgery. In his own vulgar style of humor, Green's show, live performances, book,

and cheerfully rude song all advise young men to examine them-
selves for testicular cancer. His message isn't eloquent, but it is
encouraging and upfront.

## Lance Armstrong

"If you get a second chance in life for something, go all the way,"
says Lance Armstrong. Michael Bradley's 2004 biography of this
professional bicycle athlete describes Armstrong's diagnosis of
testicular cancer in 1996 at the age of twenty-five. The cancer
had already spread to his lungs and brain, and he was given a
less than 40 percent chance of survival. But after surgery to
remove his right testicle and the brain tumors, Armstrong opted
for chemotherapy. He returned to his vigorous schedule of physical
training—often six hours each day—and recovered his strength
and endurance. Since then, he and his team of riders have won
the Tour de France seven times, and he has fathered a son and
twin daughters.

Armstrong knows that people with cancer look to him for
inspiration from their hospital rooms. He is motivated to succeed
because of their attention, and he wants to motivate them to
succeed in their own fight to survive cancer.

## Becoming a Mentor

When attending a self-help group, you'll notice after a while that
newcomers are joining. Because of your own experiences, you
might now be able to understand and give support to others who
are newly diagnosed with cancer.

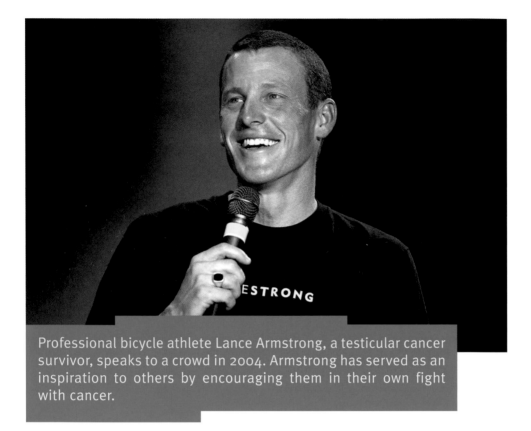

Professional bicycle athlete Lance Armstrong, a testicular cancer survivor, speaks to a crowd in 2004. Armstrong has served as an inspiration to others by encouraging them in their own fight with cancer.

You could find yourself approached by friends or acquaintances who want to have a casual conversation—or a serious one—about cancer in general or men's health concerns in particular. It can make you feel strong, experienced, and smart to help someone else find a useful Web site or learn where to get medical help. Every man who learns about the importance of self-exams is one more man participating in his own health care. You don't have to tell people every detail. Just listen to their questions, give short answers, and maybe suggest a book or a Web site.

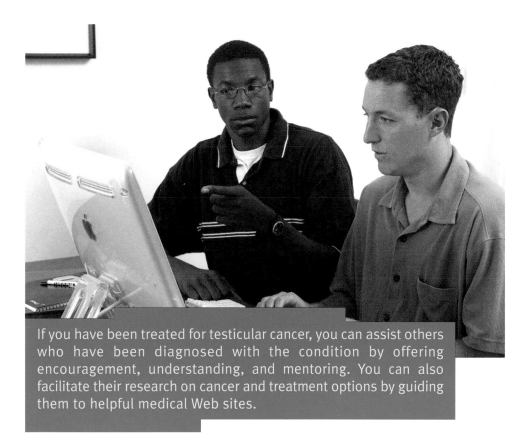

If you have been treated for testicular cancer, you can assist others who have been diagnosed with the condition by offering encouragement, understanding, and mentoring. You can also facilitate their research on cancer and treatment options by guiding them to helpful medical Web sites.

You don't have to define yourself as a cancer survivor and nothing else. You don't have to introduce yourself to everybody as a cancer survivor. You don't have to be a hero or an inspiration to everyone. But it is important to get involved in daily life and do as much as you are able, instead of avoiding ordinary responsibilities because of cancer or routine side effects from treatment.

# Glossary

**benign** A tumor that is not likely to spread.

**circumcision** Surgical removal of the prepuce (foreskin of the penis).

**epididymis** The cord that collects sperm from the testicle.

**germ cells** Cells in the testicles that make sperm.

**malignant** A tumor that is likely to grow large and spread.

**metastasized** Cancer that has spread through the body, often to the lungs, liver, or brain.

**nonseminoma** Testicular cancer, from mature (specialized) germ cells.

**orchitis** Inflammation of the testicle.

**potent** Able to have erections.

**retroperitoneal space** The anatomical space behind (retro) the abdominal cavity, notably behind the peritoneum, a membrane that covers the abdominal wall of the body.

**semen** Fluid containing sperm that is expelled during ejaculation.

**seminoma** The most common kind of testicular cancer, from immature germ cells.

**sperm** The male sex cell that is produced in the testes.

**vas deferens** The tube that takes sperm from the epididymis to the seminal vesicle.

**vasectomy** The surgical cutting and tying of the vas deferens, making a man sterile.

Helping Children Cope Program Cancer Care, Inc.
275 Seventh Avenue
New York, NY 10001
(800) 813-4673
Web site: http://www.cancercare.org
  A national nonprofit organization that provides free,
  professional support services for anyone affected by
  cancer—patient, family/friend, or health-care worker.

Kids Count, Too
American Cancer Society
15999 Clifton Road NE
Atlanta, GA 30329
(800) ACS-2345 (227-2345)
Web site: http://www.cancer.org
  An organization that provides information on surviving
  cancer of any kind, including testicular cancer. There is a
  special support group, Look Good…Feel Better for Teens,
  for cancer patients between the ages of thirteen and
  seventeen (www.2bme.org).

National Cancer Institute (NCI)
U.S. National Institutes of Health
NCI Public Inquiries Office
6116 Executive Boulevard, Room 3036A
Bethesda, MD 20892-8322
(800) 422-6237

Web site: http://www.cancer.gov
  The NCI is part of the National Institutes of Health within the
  U.S. Department of Health and Human Services. The NCI is
  the federal government's main agency for cancer research and
  training. It provides information on most kinds of cancer
  and cancer treatments.
    Assistance with navigating this detailed Web site is avail-
  able at LiveHelp, a Web site that allows typed conversations
  in real time with an information specialist who can answer
  questions about cancer, at: https://cissecure.nci.nih.gov/
  livehelp/welcome.asp.
    A fact sheet on testicular cancer is also available at:
  www.nci.nih.gov/cancertopics/factsheet/Sites-Types/testicular.

Testicular Cancer Resource Center
Web site: http://tcrc.acor.org/
  This patient-oriented Web site is written in plain language. It
  includes links to a list of testicular cancer experts your doctor
  can consult, helpful hints, humor, alternative treatments, and
  more than eighty personal stories. It offers private, individual
  e-mail support.

## Web Sites

Due to the changing nature of Internet links, Rosen Publishing
has developed an online list of Web sites related to the subject
of this book. This site is updated regularly. Please use this link
to access the list:

http://www.rosenlinks.com/faq/teca

# For Further Reading

Armstrong, Lance. *It's Not About the Bike: My Journey Back to Life.* New York, NY: Putnam, 2000.

Bradley, Michael. *Lance Armstrong* (Benchmark All-Stars). Tarrytown, NY: Marshall Cavendish, 2004.

Caldwell, Wilma R., ed. *Cancer Information for Teens: Health Tips About Cancer Awareness, Prevention, Diagnosis, and Treatment* (Teen Health Series). Detroit, MI: Omnigraphics, 2004.

Ernstoff, Marc S., ed. *Testicular and Penile Cancer.* Hanover, NH: Dartmouth Medical School, 2001.

Haylock, Pamela J., ed. *Men's Cancers: How to Prevent Them, How to Treat Them, How to Beat Them.* Alameda, CA: Hunter House, 2001.

Kenny, Paraic. *Stages of Cancer Development.* (Biology of Cancer). New York, NY: Chelsea House Publishers, 2007.

Lance Armstrong Foundation. *Live Strong: Inspirational Stories from Cancer Survivors—from Diagnosis to Treatment and Beyond.* New York, NY: Random House, 2005.

Parker, James N., and Philip M. Parker, eds. *The Official Patient's Sourcebook on Testicular Cancer. A Revised and Updated Directory for the Internet Age.* San Diego, CA: Icon Health Publications, 2002.

# Bibliography

American Cancer Society. "What Is Testicular Cancer?"
Retrieved August 5, 2006 (http://www.cancer.org/
docroot/CRI/content/CRI_2_2_1x_What_Is_Testicular_
Cancer_41.asp?sitearea=).

Armstrong, Lance. *It's Not About the Bike: My Journey
Back to Life.* New York, NY: Putnam Adult, 2000.

BC Cancer Agency. "Testes." September 2001. Retrieved
December 12, 2006 (http://www.bccancer.bc.ca/PPI/
TypesofCancer/Testes/default.htm).

Bradley, Michael. *Lance Armstrong.* Tarrytown, NY:
Marshall Cavendish, 2005.

Ernstoff, Marc S., ed. *Testicular and Penile Cancer.* Hanover,
NH: Dartmouth Medical School, 2001.

Green, Tom, and Allan Rucker. *Hollywood Causes
Cancer: The Tom Green Story.* New York, NY:
Crown, 2004.

Kantrowitz, Mark. "Testicular Cancer." Retrieved August 15,
2006 (http://www.kantrowitz.com/cancer/).

Lance Armstrong Foundation. *Livestrong: Inspirational
Stories from Cancer Survivors—From Diagnosis to
Treatment and Beyond.* New York, NY: Random
House, 2005.

Mone, Greg. "Researcher Proposes That Food Contaminant
Causes Testicular Cancer." ScientificAmerican.com.

February 4, 2002. Retrieved September 3, 2006 (http://www.sciam.com/article.cfm?articleID=00036788-E23D-1CCE-B4A8809EC588EEDF).

National Cancer Institute. "LiveHelp Service." Retrieved September 29, 2006 (https://cissecure.nci.nih.gov/livehelp/welcome.asp).

National Cancer Institute. "Testicular Cancer." Retrieved September 29, 2006 (http://www.cancer.gov/cancertopics/types/testicular).

National Cancer Institute. "Testicular Cancer: Questions and Answers." Retrieved December 11, 2006 (http://www.nci.nih.gov/cancertopics/factsheet/Sites-Types/testicular).

National Cancer Institute. "Vasectomy and Cancer Risk." June 24, 2003. Retrieved August 10, 2006 (http://www.nci.nih.gov/cancertopics/factsheet/Risk/vasectomy).

Schilling, Ray. "Testicular Cancer." Net HealthBook.com. November 21, 2006. Retrieved December 11, 2006 (http://nethealthbook.com/cancer_testicularcancer.html).

Schwartz, Gary. "What Causes Testicular Cancer?" State of the Science Web site, a project of the National Cancer Institute. December 5, 2003. Retrieved August 20, 2006 (http://www.webtie.org/sots/Meetings/Genitourinary/SUO_12_5_6_2003/transcripts/04/transcript.htm).

"Testicular Cancer." MayoClinic.com. October 3, 2005. Retrieved August 3, 2006 (http://www.mayoclinic.com/health/testicular-cancer/DS00046).

"Testicular Cancer Information and Support." Tc-Cancer.com. Retrieved August 15, 2006 (http://www.tc-cancer.com).

Testicular Cancer Resource Center. "Testicular Cancer
   Information for Everyone." November 12, 2006. Retrieved
   December 12, 2006 (http://tcrc.acor.org).
"Testicular Cancer." UrologyChannel.com. September 8, 2006.
   Retrieved December 12, 2006 (http://www.urology-channel.
   com/testicularcancer/index.shtml).
"Toxin in Certain Foods Could Cause Testicular Cancer."
   Nutraingredients.com. April 2, 2002. Retrieved August 15,
   2006 (http://www.nutraingredients.com/news/ng.asp?
   id=34373).

# Index

## Photo Credits

**Designer:** Evelyn Horovicz; **Editor**: Kathy Kuhtz Campbell
**Photo Researcher:** Marty Levick